ACUPRESSURE POINTS TO EASE ANXIETY

THE RIGHT GUIDE

A.D RAMS

Contents

CHAPTER ONE

INTRODUCTION

Acupressure is a traditional Chinese medicine (TCM)-derived ancient healing method that includes pressing on particular body spots to encourage balance and "Qi," or energy flow, in the body. Acupressure can be used in addition to medical care to help reduce anxiety symptoms, but it should never be used in place of expert medical care. An overview of certain acupressure spots that can reduce anxiety is provided here:

GV20 (Governing Vessel 20, also known as Baihui): Situated in the middle of the skull near the top of the head. This point can be stimulated to aid in mental clarity, stress reduction, and mental calmness.

HT7, also known as Shenmen or Heart 7, is a depression on the palm side of the wrist that is situated immediately below the wrist crease. By encouraging tranquility, stimulating this point may help reduce palpitations, anxiety, and insomnia.

PC6, also known as Neiguan or Pericardium 6, is situated between the two tendons and on the palm side of the forearm, three finger-widths below the wrist crease. Pushing this button can assist in reducing nausea, anxiety, and emotional imbalances.

Large Intestine 4 (LI4, also known as Hegu): Located in the webbing between the thumb and index finger on the back of the hand. It might be possible to reduce tension, headaches, and stress in the body by stimulating this spot.

Liver 3, also known as Taichong, is situated in the dip between the big and second toes on the upper part of the foot. By pushing this point, you can lessen emotional tension, encourage emotional equilibrium, and lessen impatience.

The spleen, also known as San Yin Jiao or SP6, is situated four finger-widths above the ankle bone on the inside of the leg. Activating this point could aid in mental relaxation, anxiety reduction, and improved sleep.

KD1 (Kidney 1 or Yongquan): Located on the foot sole, in the central depression beneath the ball of the foot. By applying pressure to this region, you may be able to reduce anxiety symptoms and help your body and mind relax.

Take slow, deep breaths and apply firm, mild pressure to each acupressure point for one to two minutes. It's critical to pay attention to your body and modify the pressure to a level that feels comfortable for you. You can use acupressure as a self-care technique to help manage your anxiety by including it into your daily routine, but if your anxiety symptoms are severe or chronic, you should always see a healthcare provider.

Acupuncture is an age-old medicinal practice that dates back more than 5,000 years to ancient China. It works on the same principles as acupuncture, but instead of using needles to target specific body spots, pressure is used to encourage healing, relaxation, and overall well-being.

This is a synopsis of acupressure:

The notion of Traditional Chinese Medicine (TCM), which maintains that the body's life force, or "Qi," travels along meridian routes, is the foundation of acupressure. Pain, disease, or discomfort can arise from a disruption or blockage of Qi flow. By applying pressure to particular locations along these meridians, acupressure seeks to restore Qi's flow and equilibrium.

Pressure Points: Acupressure points are found along the meridian routes on the exterior of the body. These sites are frequently located at the junctures of muscles, connective tissues, and nerves. There are hundreds of acupressure points, and each one has a unique purpose and healing impact.

Technique: To apply acupressure, press steadily on the designated spots with your fingers, thumbs, palms, or specialized tools. Depending on the person's sensitivity and the intended result, the pressure might be either light or strong. It is possible to combine the pressure with stretching or massage techniques, and it is typically applied for a few seconds to a few minutes.

Benefits: It is said that acupressure has many advantages, such as reducing stress, relieving pain, promoting relaxation, boosting immunity, improving circulation, and curing a variety of illnesses like headaches, nausea, anxiety, and sleeplessness. Acupressure is also used by some to promote spiritual development and emotional well-being.

Safety: When used appropriately, acupressure is generally safe. However, you must exercise caution when applying pressure to prevent discomfort or harm. A healthcare provider should be consulted by expectant mothers prior to using acupressure, particularly on areas that could trigger contractions. Those who have sustained specific injuries or medical disorders should also consult a licensed professional.

Integration with Modern Medicine: Although acupressure is still regarded as an adjunctive or alternative therapy, there is a growing movement to incorporate it into traditional medical settings. Acupressure is used by a wide range of healthcare providers, such as physicians, nurses, physical therapists, and massage therapists, to improve patient care and patient outcomes.

Acupressure treats the body, mind, and spirit, providing a comprehensive approach to health and wellbeing. It can be used to promote balance, relaxation, and healing as a self-care approach or as a treatment from a certified practitioner.

The Fundamentals of Acupressure

Acupressure is a conventional medical technique with roots in traditional Chinese medicine. It includes applying pressure to certain body points in order to improve health, reduce pain, and reestablish equilibrium. Here are some acupressure fundamentals:

Meridians and Qi: The foundation of acupressure is the idea of meridians, or the life force that travel through the body via channels called qi (pronounced "chee"). Traditional Chinese medicine holds that pain, sickness, and other health issues can arise from obstructed or unbalanced Qi flow. Acupressure stimulates particular meridians points in an attempt to reestablish the normal flow of Qi.

Acupressure sites: Spanning the meridians are hundreds of acupressure sites, each with specific therapeutic qualities. These spots are usually located near the confluence of muscles, connective tissues, and nerves. Applying pressure to these areas to stimulate them can help reduce stress, lessen pain, and encourage relaxation.

Techniques: Acupressure techniques apply pressure to the chosen points using fingers, thumbs, palms, elbows, or specialized equipment. Depending on the person's tolerance level and the intended result, different pressure levels might be used. Acupressure can be made more effective by using methods like kneading, stroking, tapping, and stretching in addition to direct pressure.

Benefits: It is thought that acupressure has several advantages for both mental and physical health. Pain treatment (from headaches, backaches, and menstrual cramps), stress management, relaxation, better circulation, boosted immunity, and relief from nausea, sleeplessness, and anxiety are a few of the frequently reported advantages.

Acupressure is a self-care technique that people can use to maintain their own health and well-being. They can learn how to find and activate the acupressure points on their own bodies. This can be used in conjunction with professional treatment. Furthermore, as part of a comprehensive treatment plan, it can be given by licensed practitioners including massage therapists, acupuncturists, and other medical specialists.

Safety and Precautions: When used appropriately, acupressure is generally safe, although vigilance is necessary to prevent discomfort or harm. A healthcare provider should be consulted by expectant mothers prior to using acupressure, particularly on areas that could trigger contractions. Before receiving acupressure treatment, people with certain medical issues or injuries should also consult with a trained practitioner.

In general, acupressure addresses both the physical and mental components of well-being and provides a natural, non-invasive approach to health and wellness. Acupressure, whether applied professionally or as a self-care method, can be a useful tool for fostering harmony and balance in the body.

Typical Acupressure Points to Reduce Anxiety

By encouraging relaxation, lowering stress levels, and reestablishing equilibrium in the body's energy system, acupressure can be a useful technique in the management of anxiety symptoms. The following popular acupressure spots can potentially reduce anxiety:

Governing Vessel 20 (Baihui, or GV20):

Location: In the middle of the skull, at the top of the head.

Benefits: Encouraging mental clarity, reducing tension, and calming the mind are all possible with this point stimulation.

Heart 7 or Shenmen, or HT7:

Location: In the hollow immediately below the wrist crease on the palm side of the wrist.

Benefits: Applying pressure to this spot may aid in lowering anxiety, promoting calmness, and encouraging relaxation.

PC6 (Neiguan, or Pericardium 6):

Location: Between the two tendons on the palm side of the forearm, three finger widths below the wrist crease.

Benefits: Emotional imbalances, nausea, and anxiety can all be reduced by stimulating this point.

Hegu, or Large Intestine 4, or LI4:

Location: In the webbing between the thumb and index finger on the back of the hand.

Benefits: Applying pressure to this region may help reduce tension, headaches, and stress in the body while fostering calmness.

Liver 3 (LR3, Taichong):

Location: In the space between the big and second toes on the top of the foot.

Benefits: Emotional equilibrium, reduced emotional stress, and irritation can all be achieved by stimulating this region.

Splen 6 (also known as San Yin Jiao):

Location: Four finger-widths above the ankle bone on the inside of the leg.

Benefits: Applying pressure to this spot may aid in mental clarity, lower anxiety, and enhance sleep quality.

Kidney 1 or Yongquan, or KD1:

Location: In the center of the depression beneath the foot's ball, on the sole of the foot.

Benefits: Activating this point may assist reduce anxiety symptoms, quiet the mind, and help the body ground.

Use your fingertips or thumbs to apply light to hard pressure to these acupressure points. To improve relaxation, hold each point for one to two minutes while inhaling deeply and slowly. It's critical to pay attention to your body and modify the pressure to a level that feels comfortable for you. You can use acupressure as a self-care technique to help manage your anxiety by including it into your daily routine, but if your anxiety symptoms are severe or chronic, you should always see a healthcare provider.

Methodologies for Using Acupressure

Acupressure can be applied in a variety of ways, each with its own advantages and methods for enhancing health and wellbeing. Here are a few typical methods for using acupressure:

Direct Force:

This is the simplest method; all you have to do is use your fingertips, thumb, or palm to apply consistent pressure directly to the acupressure point.

For one to two minutes, apply strong yet mild pressure to the location, adjusting the pressure progressively to suit your comfort level.

Applying direct pressure can help release tension, encourage relaxation, and reduce pain.

Rotating Motion:

Using your fingertips or thumbs, apply circular motion to the acupressure point in place of static pressure.

Start by lightly pressing the spot in a clockwise or counterclockwise circular motion.

As you continue the circular motion, gradually apply more pressure, paying particular attention to any sore spots or regions of stress.

In addition to promoting relaxation and releasing muscle tension, circular motion can aid increase blood flow.

CHAPTER TWO

Kneading:

This method entails kneading or massaging the acupressure point and its environs with your fingers or thumbs.

Like you would while kneading dough, apply light pressure and start kneading the area in a circular manner.

As necessary, gradually apply more pressure, paying particular attention to tense or painful areas.

Kneading can promote relaxation, increase circulation, and aid release knots in the muscles.

Drumming or Schlagwerk:

Using your fingertips or a soft object to lightly touch the acupressure point and its surroundings is known as tapping or percussion.

For thirty to sixty seconds, tap the point rhythmically with a light yet quick tapping stroke.

Tapping has the potential to increase energy flow, energize the body, and facilitate relaxation.

Extending

To increase their efficacy, several acupressure sites can be used in conjunction with stretching methods.

Stimulate the acupressure point and stretch the muscles or body part nearby at the same time.

Hold the stretch while applying pressure to the acupressure point for approximately 30 to 1 minute.

Stretching aids in stress relief, increased flexibility, and relaxation.

Breathing Techniques:

When used with acupressure, deep breathing techniques can help induce relaxation and peace.

Breathe in deeply and slowly through your nose to expand your abdomen. Breathe out slowly through your mouth to release tension with each breath.

Breathe in as you apply pressure and out as you release pressure when using the acupressure techniques.

It's crucial to pay attention to your body when using acupressure techniques and modify the pressure and intensity according to how comfortable you are. As needed, progressively raise the pressure while being careful not to inflict pain or discomfort. Start with less force. To support general health and wellbeing, acupressure can be routinely used as part of a self-care regimen.

A Comprehensive Guide for Acupressure Treatments

This is a detailed tutorial on how to run an acupressure session:

Set Up Your Area:

Locate a peaceful, cozy area where you may unwind without being bothered.

To create a relaxing atmosphere, make sure there is enough lighting and ventilation.

To access the acupressure points you intend to work on, find a comfortable position to sit or lie down comfortably.

Decide on Your Goals:

Establish your intentions for the acupressure session in a moment. This could be relieving pain, reducing tension, relaxing, or achieving any other particular objective you have in mind.

As the session starts, picture yourself in a state of balance, calmness, and relaxation.

Acupressure Point Identification:

Depending on your unique requirements or objectives, choose which acupressure points to focus on. To find the points that pertain to your concerns, consult a chart or guide.

The points you select should match the symptoms or trouble spots you are experiencing.

Put Some Pressure On It:

Apply consistent pressure to the chosen acupressure sites using your fingertips, thumb, palm, or a specialized acupressure tool.

Don't use too much force; instead, start out gently and increase as necessary.

Try out a variety of methods, including tapping, kneading, direct pressure, circular motion, and stretching, to see which ones are most comfortable and productive for you.

Concentrate on your breathing:

Align your breathing with the acupressure points to improve energy flow and relaxation.

Breathe in deeply and slowly through your nose to expand your abdomen. Breathe out slowly through your mouth to release tension with each breath.

Throughout the practice, keep your breathing rhythm calm and consistent.

Retain Every Point:

Apply consistent pressure to each acupressure point for a duration of one to two minutes, or longer if preferred.

At each point, concentrate on the feelings that come over you, such as warmth, tingling, or relaxation.

Proceed in Sequence:

When working on several acupressure points at once, proceed methodically and sequentially from one point to the next.

Before going on to the following point, give each one careful thought and attention.

Pay Attention to Your Body:

Observe how your body reacts to the acupressure methods.

If you feel pain or discomfort, modify the pressure or method or, if required, stop applying pressure to that location.

Wrap Up the Meeting:

Release pressure from each acupressure point gradually after you have treated all of the desired points or reached your desired result.

Give yourself a few minutes to rest and unwind so that the acupressure's effects can fully take hold in your body.

Think and Drink:

Think back for a moment on your feelings following the acupressure session. Observe any alterations in your emotional, mental, or physical health.

To stay hydrated and aid the body's natural healing processes, sip on a glass of water.

Keep in mind that when using acupressure, consistency is essential. Over time, consistent attendance might result in cumulative advantages. Before beginning an acupressure practice, it is always a good idea to speak with a skilled healthcare provider if you have any specific health concerns or conditions.

Complementary Methods for Reducing Anxiety

Several complementary therapies, in addition to acupressure, can lessen anxiety and enhance general wellbeing. Here are a few useful complementary techniques to reduce anxiety:

Meditation with mindfulness:

During mindfulness meditation, one practices nonjudgmental present-moment awareness. By encouraging relaxation, raising self-awareness, and fostering serenity, it helps lessen anxiety.

Anxiety management techniques including body scans, loving-kindness meditation, and mindful breathing can be especially helpful.

Breathing Techniques:

Exercises that involve deep breathing can assist trigger the body's relaxation response, which lowers stress and anxiety levels. To encourage serenity and relaxation, practice breathing exercises like 4-7-8 breathing, diaphragmatic breathing, and alternate nostril breathing on a daily basis.

Yoga:

Yoga encourages relaxation, flexibility, and mental clarity through a combination of physical postures, breathing exercises, and meditation. Regular yoga practice can help lessen the symptoms of anxiety by promoting a sense of well-being, relieving tension, and boosting circulation.

Yoga nidra (guided relaxation), moderate flow sequences, and restorative yoga are very helpful in reducing anxiety.

PMR, or progressive muscle relaxation, is:

To relieve stress and encourage relaxation, PMR entails methodically tensing and relaxing various body muscular groups. This method can assist in easing the tightness and tension in the muscles that are indicative of anxiety.

Online guided PMR sessions can be used on a regular basis to help reduce symptoms of anxiety.

Aromatherapy:

Using essential oils made from plants, aromatherapy helps people unwind and feel less anxious. A few relaxing essential oils, including bergamot, lavender, and chamomile, can be inhaled, used topically, or diffused to help reduce the symptoms of anxiety.

For maximum benefit, aromatherapy can be coupled with other methods of relaxation like deep breathing or meditation.

Practice:

Regular exercise that releases endorphins (feel-good hormones) and encourages relaxation, such walking, jogging, cycling, or dancing, can help lower anxiety.

Try to get in at least 30 minutes of moderate-to-intense exercise most days of the week to reap the benefits of exercise on your mood.

Writing a Journal:

Keeping a journal can be a useful tool for understanding anxiety patterns, recognizing triggers, and processing feelings. Rumination can be lessened and self-awareness can be increased by putting your ideas, feelings, and experiences in writing.

To control anxiety and develop a good outlook, try journaling exercises like free writing, gratitude journaling, or reflection journaling.

Herbal Treatments:

Herbal medicines have long been used to ease anxiety and encourage relaxation. Some of these cures include valerian root, passionflower, and chamomile.

Before utilizing herbal medicines, especially if you have any underlying health concerns or are taking medication, consult with a trained healthcare expert or herbalist.

CBT, or cognitive-behavioral therapy:

Cognitive behavioral therapy (CBT) is a type of psychotherapy that aims to alter unfavorable cognitive patterns and anxiety-related behaviors. It can support people in overcoming illogical beliefs, constructing resilience, and learning coping mechanisms.

Working with a qualified counselor or therapist can offer individualized assistance and direction for using CBT approaches to manage anxiety.

Social Assistance:

Reducing emotions of loneliness and isolation, which are frequent anxiety triggers, can be accomplished by upholding strong social relationships and asking friends, family, or support groups for assistance.

When you're stressed or anxious, reach out to people you can trust for emotional support, motivation, and company.

When these complimentary techniques are combined with acupressure, a holistic strategy for reducing anxiety and enhancing general wellbeing can be developed. Try out a range of methods to see which one suits you the best, and for best outcomes, think about implementing many habits into your everyday schedule. Furthermore, it's critical to get expert assistance from a healthcare physician or mental health professional if your anxiety symptoms are severe or ongoing.

Advantages and Things to Think About When Using Acupressure for Anxiety

Acupuncture for anxiety has many advantages, but before adding it to your wellness regimen, there are a few things you should know. Here are some advantages and things to think about:

Advantages:

Natural Relaxation: By stimulating particular body points, acupressure helps promote relaxation and ease tension, both of which can help lessen the symptoms of anxiety.

Stress Reduction: This technique can help quiet the mind and lessen the physiological consequences of stress on the body by focusing on acupressure points linked to stress alleviation.

Non-Invasive: Acupressure is a non-invasive alternative to acupuncture that many people find more comfortable and accessible because it does not require the use of needles.

Self-Care strategy: Acupressure is a practical self-care strategy for daily anxiety management because it is simple to perform at home.

Complementary Approach: Acupressure can increase the efficacy of other anxiety-reduction methods by working in tandem with mindfulness, relaxation, and treatment.

Holistic wellbeing: Acupressure offers a comprehensive approach to wellbeing since it is based on holistic concepts, which take into account the interdependence of the body, mind, and spirit.

Taking into account

Individual Variability: Since everyone reacts to acupressure differently, what works well for one person might not have the same impact on another. It's critical to try out various methods and strategies to determine which ones work best for you.

Expert Advice: Although acupressure can be used on its own, it is best to get advice from a licensed acupressure practitioner or healthcare provider to ensure safe and efficient administration, particularly if you have any underlying health issues.

Like with any fitness regimen, frequent practice and consistency are essential to reaping the full advantages of acupressure for anxiety alleviation. It could require persistence and patience to notice appreciable adjustments in anxiety symptoms.

Severity of Symptoms: For mild to moderate anxiety symptoms, acupressure may be more beneficial. It's critical to speak with a healthcare provider about comprehensive treatment options for severe or chronic anxiety, as they may involve counseling, medication, or other interventions.

Safety precautions: Although acupressure is generally safe, it should be used carefully to prevent pain or harm.

CHAPTER THREE

Acupressure should not be applied by pregnant women without first consulting a healthcare professional and employing caution, especially on sites that could cause contractions.

Integration with Other Therapies: Acupressure can be used in conjunction with other anxiety treatments. However, it's important to let your healthcare provider know about any complementary methods you're using on a regular basis.

All things considered, acupressure can be a useful technique for reducing anxiety and enhancing general wellbeing, but it's important to use caution, patience, and regard for each person's unique requirements and circumstances while using it. Acupressure is an age-old therapeutic technique that can potentially relieve anxiety for those who incorporate it within a holistic approach to wellness.

Applications in Real Life and Case Studies

Case studies and real-world applications offer insightful information about how well acupressure works to relieve anxiety. Although acupressure is still undergoing scientific investigation, case studies and anecdotal data provide strong indications of its possible advantages. Here are a few case studies and real-world applications:

1. Self-Healing Techniques:

Many people use acupressure as part of their regular self-care regimens to treat their anxiety symptoms. For instance, someone who is stressed out at work could apply acupressure techniques to ease tension and encourage relaxation during breaks.

These self-care techniques can involve deep breathing exercises, applying pressure to particular acupressure spots, or utilizing acupressure in mindfulness meditation sessions.

2. Integrated Medical Environments:

A holistic approach to treating anxiety in hospital settings frequently includes the use of acupressure. For those with anxiety disorders, for example, a mental health center might provide acupuncture and acupressure in addition to counseling and medication.

In these situations, acupressure can be combined with other therapies to treat anxiety's psychological as well as physical components.

3. Case Studies:

Case studies include in-depth descriptions of real-world acupressure experiences for the reduction of anxiety. A case study could explain, for instance, how a person with generalized anxiety disorder (GAD) used acupressure methods to treat symptoms including tense muscles, restlessness, and excessive worry.

These case studies frequently show improvements in anxiety symptoms, including decreased panic episode frequency and intensity, better sleep, and increased general wellbeing.

4. Community-Oriented Initiatives:

Acupressure workshops or classes may be included in community-based programs and wellness initiatives to teach people how to utilize acupressure for anxiety self-management.

These programs include instruction, tools, and practical training in acupressure techniques, and they may be tailored to particular demographics, such as students, the elderly, or people who suffer from chronic stress.

5. Online Sources and Communities of Support:

People can use internet forums, blogs, and social media groups as platforms to discuss their experiences using acupressure to relieve anxiety.

Users can exchange success stories, talk about their preferred acupressure points and methods, and support and encourage those who are looking for all-natural anxiety solutions.

Although these case studies and real-world examples offer encouraging proof of the potential advantages of acupressure for anxiety reduction, it's important to evaluate them cautiously. Because it is subjective, anecdotal evidence might not accurately reflect the experiences of all people. Furthermore, more thorough studies—such as systematic reviews and randomized controlled trials—are required to determine whether acupressure is beneficial for treating anxiety in a range of contexts and demographics.

Seeking Expert Advice and Assistance

It is imperative that anyone considering utilizing acupressure or any complementary therapy for anxiety management obtain professional advice and assistance. Here's why it matters and some advice on how to approach it:

The Value of Expert Counseling:

Safety: Although acupressure is typically safe, doing it incorrectly might cause pain or damage. Acupressure is the application of pressure to certain places on the body. Advice on safe procedures and techniques can be given by a licensed professional.

Effectiveness: Skilled acupressure practitioners know how to choose the right spots and techniques based on each client's unique needs. Personalized recommendations can be provided by them depending on your medical history and particular symptoms.

Integration with Conventional Treatment: It's important to talk to your healthcare practitioner about complementary therapies like acupressure if you're currently receiving therapy or medication for anxiety. They can assist in making sure that acupressure doesn't conflict with other therapies and instead enhances your current treatment plan.

Progress Monitoring: An experienced practitioner can keep an eye on your development over time and modify your acupressure treatment regimen as necessary. They can also offer you continuing support and direction to help you reach your objectives.

How to Look for Expert Advice:

Locate a Qualified Practitioner: Seek out acupressure professionals who have undergone official training and certification in either acupressure or traditional Chinese medicine (TCM). You can look up listings online, consult medical professionals for advice, or ask friends or relatives for recommendations.

Investigate Credentials: Find out about a practitioner's background, education, and experience. Select an acupuncturist or acupressure practitioner who is licensed, certified, or registered with a reputable professional organization.

Make an Appointment: Set up a meeting with the practitioner to go about your expectations, goals, and worries related to using acupressure to relieve anxiety. Take advantage of this chance to share pertinent health information, ask questions, and voice any reservations or requests you may have.

Observe Recommendations: The practitioner may suggest particular acupressure sites, techniques, and the number of sessions based on your consultation and needs. Throughout the course of treatment, heed their advice and voice any criticism or concerns.

Keep Up: Remain aware of the advantages, dangers, and restrictions surrounding the use of acupressure for the treatment of anxiety. To gain a deeper grasp of the discipline, ask the practitioner for resources, instructional materials, or recommendations to reliable sources of information.

Talk to Your Healthcare Team: Tell your physician that you have chosen to include acupressure in your anxiety treatment regimen. They can offer advice, keep an eye on your development, and make sure acupressure complements your overall medical objectives.

You can improve the safety, efficacy, and general experience of utilizing acupressure as a supplemental therapy for anxiety alleviation by getting expert advice and assistance. You can be confident that you will receive individualized care and direction that is specific to your requirements and situation when you work with a skilled practitioner.

Summary

In conclusion, by encouraging relaxation, lowering stress levels, and reestablishing equilibrium within the body's energy system, acupressure presents a viable strategy for treating anxiety. This age-old therapeutic method, which has its roots in traditional Chinese medicine, includes pressing on particular body locations to promote energy flow and reduce anxiety symptoms.

Acupressure can help relieve stress, soothe the mind, and enhance wellbeing by using light pressure and a variety of techniques include circular motion, kneading, tapping, and stretching. Regular acupressure treatments can enhance other anxiety-reduction techniques including mindfulness, deep breathing exercises, yoga, and cognitive-behavioral therapy when included in a holistic approach to wellness.

Acupressure may help reduce anxiety, according to case studies and anecdotal evidence, but it's important to approach the practice mindfully, patiently, and with care for each patient's unique needs. Application safety and efficacy can be ensured by seeking professional advice and assistance from licensed acupressure practitioners or healthcare experts, particularly for individuals with underlying health disorders or concerns.

Along with other complementary therapies and traditional medical interventions, a comprehensive self-care regimen that includes acupressure can enable people to actively participate in managing their anxiety and enhancing their general well-being. A natural and approachable technique to attain balance and serenity in the face of life's obstacles, acupressure promotes a holistic approach to health that takes into account the body, mind, and spirit.

THE END